AF255860

JOIN A HEALTH REVOLUTION

7 STEPS TO A HEALTHIER YOU

THE SECRET TO HOW SIMPLE NUTRITION LEADS TO A HEALTHY YOU!

LU CREWS

JOIN A HEALTH REVOLUTION!

7 STEPS TO A

HEALTHIER

YOU

THE SECRET TO HOW SIMPLE NUTRITION LEADS TO A HEALTHY YOU!

LU CREWS, HEALTH ADVOCATE

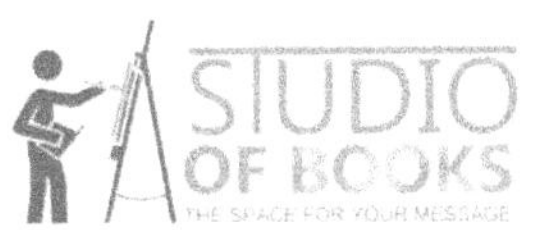

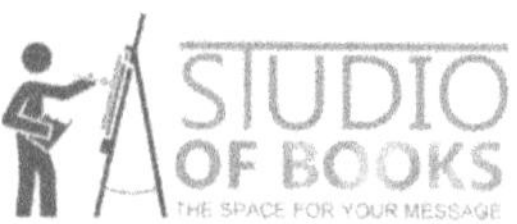

Copyright © 2025 by Lu Crews

All rights reserved. No part of this publication may be reproduced, distributed, or transmitted in any form or by any means, including photocopying, recording, or other electronic or mechanical methods, without the prior written permission of the copyright owner and the publisher, except in the case of brief quotations embodied in critical reviews and certain other noncommercial uses permitted by copyright law. For permission requests, write to the publisher, "Attention: Permissions Coordinator," to the address below.

Studio of Books LLC
5900 Balcones Drive Suite 100
Austin, Texas 78731
www.studioofbooks.org
Hotline: (254) 800-1183

Ordering Information:
Special discounts are available on quantity purchases by corporations, associations, and others. For details, contact the publisher at the address above.

Printed in the United States of America.

ISBN-13: Softcover   978-1-964928-25-8
          eBook   978-1-964928-26-5

Library of Congress Control Number: 2025904587

DISCLAIMER

The information in this book is provided for informational purposes only and is not a substitute for professional medical advice or the services of a physician. The author and publisher make no legal claims, express or implied, and the material is not intended to replace the diagnosis or treatment of a disease.

The author, publisher and/or copyright holder assume no responsibility for the loss or damage caused, or allegedly caused, directly or indirectly by the use of information contained in this book. The author and publisher specially disclaim any liability incurred from the use or application of the contents of this book.

Throughout this book rather than putting a trademark symbol in every occurrence of a trademarked name, we state that we are using names and information in an editorial fashion only and to the benefit of the trademark owner and no intention of infringement of the trademark.

First Edition, 2015

DEDICATION

This book is dedicated to Donald Mayfield, NMD, DOM (1937-2015) whose brilliant mind taught me the holistic principles of healing. There were others that followed, but he was the first and the most important in that aspect of my life teachings.

Also to my family, late husband Donald, my daughters Christine (Gerry) and Cathleen (Ken) and my sons Donny (Mai) and Tommy. I thank them for putting up with their mother's sometimes weird ways, and for their carrying on the tradition of holistic healing.

A special thanks to Christine and Cathleen for their willingness to read through and patiently critique my manuscript.

And I must thank the Holy Spirit who gave me the vision for this book.

Brig Hart, R3GTeam
Lita Hart, R3GTeam

PREFACE

To say I am proud of my Mother, my mentor and my best friend is an understatement! Lu Crews, Mother, has been an inspiration to thousands of people over her many years on this planet. She has a divine inspiration from God to herald the very worthy message of a healthy & more prosperous life. When I say at my speaking engagements that 'She pioneered a health revolution', I mean it. She was always first to push the envelope and question "why?" Why are artificial ingredients necessary in this…? Why is a mother's own milk not the perfect food for her own baby? Why have a soda machine on a middle school campus? Why let some man tell her what to feed her children. She always thought outside – of – the – box when it came to our family's health and has instilled that same spirit in myself.

I strongly urged my Mother to write this book, and more to come. I know this is her legacy. As the great, late mentor, Miles Monroe so eloquently states, " Where are the greatest masterpieces, the most glorious songs or the best words ever written? Where are these gems held? The grave yard…for in it are all the ideas, vision and thoughts that never came to bless us!" Our legacy is meant to be shared now and I am grateful this book is here in print.

So, I acknowledge and thank my Mother, Lu for putting this work together and I strongly encourage her to continue to bless us with her true gift of health and the desire for a better way…

Christine Crews O'Shea

TESTIMONIALS

"Lu Crews has always been ahead of her time, providing a wealth of knowledge in options for self-care, healing and optimum health. Once again we are called to action, remaining pro-active and taking the next steps to smart living. Lu has provided a user-friendly step by step tool for self-healing in today's modern lifestyle."

DawnCastillo, Program Advisor for Soul of Yoga Institute, Encinitas, CA

"Lu has indirectly influenced our life through her daughter Christine O'Shea. It has been a huge blessing in my family's journey to be partnered with her family. I can't wait to read Lu's new book."

Kelli Bono, Health Advocate

"I have known Lu for 50+ years. I am one of those friends that didn't get her at first – but over the years she has stirred my interest into living a healthy lifestyle."

Janice Castillo, Friend

"Lu has been a special friend for a good many years. In all the years her passion has always been enlightening people how to take an active role in their health and nutrition. I was one of those friends who thought she was way out there. But through her patience and caring I came from being a pepsi and snicker candy bar guy, to an advocate in living a heathy lifestyle."

BrigHart, Evolv Health Products

"I am excited about Lu writing a book. Though all the years I have known her she has been sharing her knowledge about health and nutrition. I for one, am grateful that through her sharing she was able to help me turn my life around when I was very ill. I am thankful that through learning from her, I too, am able to now share with others what it means to focus on holistic healing and good sound nutrition."

Lita Hart, Evolv Health Products

"Lu has written a comprehensive guide to help people progress from where they are health wise, to where they need to be. Although I have personally known Lu for a few years, she was mentored by the same man, Dr. Donald Mayfield, as my dad, Dr. Dan Clark, and crossed paths many years ago."

Dr. Dana Clark-McGrady, AP, DOM Better Health &
Wellness Center

TABLE OF CONTENTS

STAYING POSITIVE LEADS TO GOOD HEALTH

This Book has been written with one purpose in mind: to help and inspire that person who wants to change not only how they eat, but their lifestyle. My purpose was not to write a technical book, but a book outlining easy to follow steps to a healthy you. My intention is to present in a concise manner what I have learned over the many years of studying health and nutrition.

BALANCE 1

WHY A REVOLUTION – MY STORY

"True healthcare starts in your home, not in Washington"

Anonymous

Revolution!! What does it mean when I say, "Do you want to be a part of a health revolution?"

Revolution is defined in the dictionary as:

(1) a far-reaching or drastic change;

(2) one complete turn;

(3) a cycle of successive events or change; and

(4) a profound change in conditions.

The synonyms for revolution are:

(1) revolt;

(2) rebellion;

(3) transformation; and

(4) rejection.

What I am referring to here is a peaceful revolution, where bold, courageous, reliable people work together to bring change.

All these definitions could be used for what I have been doing for the last fifty years!

My Story. This is not my first revolution. To give you background, I need to go back to my high school years when I would hand out pamphlets to my friends who had just begun to smoke, on how smoking could cause cancer. Not a popular stand to take with teenagers just beginning to defy their parents. I also would not allow my friends to smoke in my car. Fast forward many years, I was the unpopular mother who had chocolate milk taken out of the elementary school my children were attending, providing research showing that the added sugar led to ADD and other behavioral problems.

The Beginning. My revolution really began in early 1960, before I had children. My husband and I had just gotten out of college. I knew I wanted to have children, and with my "need to know" personality, I started to do research on natural childbirth. I was convinced this is what I wanted to do. I had already read Adelle Davis' book Let's Get Well, a woman ahead of her time in the nutrition field. I knew I wanted the best for my family.

I become certified to be a Lazame trainer. Lazame is a system of teaching a natural, healthy, and safe approach to pregnancy, childbirth and early parenting.

I also did research on breastfeeding and knew this is what I would do. Since there was no one around to coach me, I decided I would learn enough so I could teach classes and therefore be confident in what I was doing when the time came. I got my certification to hold classes for pregnant woman and then would council with new mothers on the joy of breastfeeding. I obtained my certification from the LaLeche League, a group of forward thinking young woman out of Franklin Park, Illinois. They are a non-profit organization dedicated to providing information, support, education, and encouragement to woman who want the best for their children and families. As it turned out, for a good many years, I touched many wonderful young women's lives and made drastic changes in their way of thinking about childbirth, health and nutrition. My reward came twenty years later when the daughters of my friends came to me wanting to experience natural childbirth and breastfeeding.

Why do I consider this a revolution? You have to understand what the norm was for giving birth in the 1960's. Standard procedure was to administer a gas-scopolamine which caused a twilight sleep. More often than not, woman had nasty reactions and some would hallucinate, often needing to be physically restrained. This is true as barbaric as it sounds. This was because the drug did not reduce the pain, but instead induced a state of disorientation. Dad's were relegated to the waiting room so as not to witness the awful side effects of the procedure. This also produced very drugged up babies as the drugs do pass thru to the placenta. This caused problems in trying to nurse, because these newborn babies were not responsive to nursing. As far as breastfeeding went, you were strictly on your own.

When I started out on this revolution, my intention was to help change the thinking about childbirth for woman and doctors and hospitals. Childbirth is not a medical issue, but a very natural phenomena. I wanted to change how woman were treated by doctors who gave them no control or information over what was happening in their bodies. I remember that one of the doctors I was seeing called me a fanatic when I told him I wanted to have a natural birth with no drugs. He refused to see me again.

Most of the time after giving birth, women were not allowed out of bed for four or five days. I was up immediately After giving birth, actually assisting and encouraging a new mother nurse her newborn in the hospital. This woman, whom I did not know at the time, is still a friend after 47 years. Actually this little baby boy three years later, became my son's best friend as still is.

I remember one of the women in my natural childbirth class who was told by her mother that childbirth was like "walking through the valley of death!" Consequently as a result of learning the true nature of childbirth, she had a beautiful delivery with three children and her daughter also carried on the tradition. Even if the women who came to my class did not want to go through childbirth without drugs, I taught them that what was happening to their bodies was natural, not something to be frightened of.

My Experiences. I not only taught, but I practiced it. My first pregnancy was a disaster! My doctor was a clueless old man who had no idea what I wanted to do, nor did he have a desire to accommodate me with my wishes. My second pregnancy, was better, I was able to convince the doctor I meant what I said about having a natural delivery. By mu third pregnancy, I had the opportunity to teach and educate some of the medical professionals in my area the long term benefits of rooming in and natural childbirth. The advantage in rooming in is having the baby in your room and not in the nursery, therefore being able to nurse him/her when they were hungry, not having to wait for a scheduled feeding determined by the hospital, not by the baby. Natural childbirth eliminates the drugs used in a medicated birth, from entering the baby. I was actually the first (and second, two years later), to have rooming in at Wuesthoff Hospital in Rockledge.

I took my campaign to whoever would listen. I was fortunate to be allowed to teach a group of young woman in nursing program at our local college about natural childbirth and breast feeding, something that was not being taught at the time. Of course there were many who were not ready to listen. I was called an extremist by many, but I wore that title as a badge of honor.

My Journey. I also was on a journey of helping people realize what they were eating had a big impact on how they were feeling. I was taking classes at a naturopathic college and also learning from several holistic doctors. I was more interested in holistic healing versus using drugs to mask the real reason behind sickness and disease. I am not against the medical profession, but believe there is a place for those of us who want to go about healing in a more natural way.

In the late 70's aspartame was introduced to the world. A group of us concerned parents had been following the research on this new "sugar substitute." We had read the reports on the concerns of a group of scientist that this "toxic waste product", and that is what it really was, could be harmful to the brain cells that affect memory, children being particularly susceptible. The reports were there to read, but the FDA approved the use of this chemical, and there was no stopping the release of this "new" replacement for sugar. More on this in a later chapter.

Who were my followers? During the 1960's I was conducting seminars and gathering a following, but I realized most of my followers were the real fringe in society. These women were burning their bras in protest (this is true) making a statement for equal rights, but I was educating them to take a stand. But I just could not seem to break through to the mom and dads who I was trying to reach. Even my close friends, at that time, were very skeptical of my beliefs and teachings. Eventually they would come around to recognize that I had something positive to offer, and I had many convert to healthy eating and alternative health care. I became "Dr. Lu" to many who would come to me for advice on "what should I do if…" I have been blessed with a desire to know, not one who would take someone's word on any given subject.

A Cycle of Change. So why a revolution? As one dictionary defines it – "A cycle of successive events or changes." I believe we are in that cycle right now. Never before have I experienced so many people wanting to take charge of their own and their family's health, not relying on the "opinion" of so many doctors who unfortunately only know how to rely on the pharmaceutical companies and their bottom line. I know there are doctors who are willing to look at the alternatives available. Actually more and more are coming on the bandwagon because that is what their patients want. Drugs have their place, particularly when involving emergency situations and broken bones, but please, let me and my family make our own informed decisions on methods to treat whatever health challenges we are facing.

We are not in a bubble. As I have stated before, we are in the middle of a cycle of change, sometimes not so good, but the health awareness cycle of change is for the good. I have to mention a couple of organizations that are fueling this change.

The Million Mom Movement. This group is headed by a lady named Amy Venner. To quote her mission statement; We're on a mission to help one million families eat cleaner and greener. Dave Sandoval (founder of Purium) has been sounding the warning against the processed foods industry for more than two decades. Now we have a game plan, a blueprint and a specific goal to put this vision into action. I am so proud of what this Million Mom Movement could mean for the health of our country and the world. Dave and I won't stop until the goal has been reached and we are one million strong! My daughter Christine introduced this movement to me. Balance 3 goes into detail of what it means to eat cleaner and greener. I will discuss this more in depth in subsequent chapters.

Moms Across America. MAA is a national coalition of unstoppable moms whose mottos is: *Empowerment Moms, Healthy Kids*. Their organization's intention is to raise awareness and support Moms with solutions to eat GMO (genetically modified organisms) free as we demand GMO labelling locally and nationally simultaneously. I will go into this more in a later chapter. My daughter, Cathleen recently was in a march sponsored by the MAA.

My Heritage. Speaking of daughters, I am blessed to have two daughters both whom are strong advocates of everything I stand for. They both had natural childbirth, my oldest daughter, Christine, having two children.

Christine has been in lock-step with me on eating healthy. She is the one who encouraged me to write this book. She has been a great help in reading and critiquing these pages as I write. Christine, from a very young age, took up her mother's banner on eating healthy. From the time she was 10 years old, she was in the kitchen with me anxious to learn. Her children have also been raised with a focus on healthy eating. Her son, David, wrote a paper for his college health class and speech class on the dangers of artificial sweeteners. Jessica, her daughter, is a vegetarian. Christine is an active promoter, spokesperson and leader in the health movement today. She is taking the message of creating healthy living for families across the country.

Cathleen, my youngest daughter, has seven children and all by natural childbirth. The last one was a home birth with her 18 years old daughter, Hannah Lu, assisting the mid-wife! Cathleen is a home school Mom and her children have been learning about healthy living from a very young age. Scripture says; "train up your child in the way they should go and they will not depart from you." She too is a spokesperson for a healthy lifestyle. Cathleen and her family live on a farm where they have free range chickens, grass feed cattle, pigs, and a wonderful organic garden. The tradition marches on.

I am very blessed to have both my daughters share my passion and take up my "revolution" in helping to change people's attitudes on healthy living.

Both my sons are strong in the nutrition aspects of healthy eating, also. My oldest son, Donny, always seemed to follow in my footsteps by enjoying healthy foods. In the last couple of years Donny has planted an "urban garden," in the backyard of his Denver home. He grows beautiful organic vegetables, in the summer of course. I guess it comes by him naturally, my dad always had a garden. He even has chickens in his Denver backyard! He called me very excited when he got his first eggs.

My youngest son, Tommy, never seemed to be interested in what he was eating. Although all was not lost on him. I realized it when I got a call from his high school principal that Tommy was causing trouble in one of his classes. This was not new for Tommy, he always seemed to lead the pack when pranks were happening. This time he got trouble because he corrected the home economics teacher when she was explaining about nutrition and Tommy stood up and said, "No that is not correct, my mom teaches..." So Tommy was listening and learning even when I did not think so. He too, is now a strong advocate for healthy living.

So this is my story. I pray as you read through my book, you will be inspired to take up your own "revolution" by breaking though old eating patterns, and by taking the responsibility to change your health and the health of your family. I will be talking about the other "fronts" in this revolution, which I will be going into as we progress through this book. So march on!

Lu Crews

BALANCE 2

IMPORTANCE OF KEEPING AN ALKALINE/ACID ENVIRONMENT IN YOUR BODY

"a peaceful heart leads to a healthy body;

jealousy is like cancer to the bones"

Proverbs 14:30

Important Information. This is not a subject that I would say would excite anyone. But none the less, it is important to learn about this aspect of your health. It is very basic to your health.

Challenges. I will start with this first because it has become of epidemic proportions in our society, indigestion and acid reflux. Acid reflux is basically acid indigestion or what we used to call, heartburn. It is very uncomfortable for people that experience it and I am not making light of it. The drugs such as Nexium, Prilosec or Prevacid and the over the counter tablets like Tums and Rolaids actually make this condition worse. Acid reflux is actually a symptom, not a disease, and the medical profession is totally missing the mark of what is the root cause and how it is being treated. Actually using acid reducing drugs adds to this problem by decreasing the acid in your stomach, where it is needed to break down our food. This is counterproductive to the acid reflux you are suffering. I know it is frustrating to hear another drug is doing terrible things to your body.

Consequences of Low Stomach Acid. Did you know that approximately 90% of Americans have low stomach acid? Low stomach acid leads to a cascade of problems. Here are some of the consequences of using acid inhibitors to lower your stomach acid for your acid reflux.

- Low stomach acid cannot properly break down proteins into amino acids.

- Low stomach acid fosters imbalanced gut flora. Lack of acidity in the stomach makes it more hospitable to unhealthy bacterial growth.

- Low stomach acid leads to nutrient malabsorption. We need our stomach acid to break down our foods so that our bodies can absorb the nutrients.

- Low stomach acid leads to heartburn/GERD/reflux as demonstrated above.

- Low stomach acid often means constipation, bloating, gas and belching. With inadequate acid, food sits in the stomach and putrefies instead of being properly digested.

- Low stomach acid may cause leaky gut and therefore create allergies.

Heartburn Drugs. You may have seen the headlines recently about how heartburn frugs increase you risk of heart attacks by about 15% to 20%. This is the conclusion of a new study by Dr. Nigam H. Shah of Stanford University. Heartburn drugs called *proton pump inhibitors*, block the production of nitric oxide, causing your blood vessels to become stiff and narrow. This leads to a lack of oxygen. Nitric oxide is something you need more of, not less of. Also as we age our bodies naturally makes less nitric oxide and that is a problem in itself. Depending it with drugs has serious consequences.

Natural Cause, Natural Cure. Actually, let's talk about what causes this symptom and what this chapter is all about, having an acid environment in your body. One of the major causes of acid reflux is the consumption of refined sugar and refined grains. Eliminating any acid ash producing food will give sufferers relief. Also stress will sometimes cause the esophageal sphincter which is supposed to close after you eat, but stress will sometimes causes it to stay open. This happens in the minority of acid reflux. This means changing the way you eat and what you eat will give acid reflux sufferers relief, which is what this whole "revolution" is all about – changing the habits that are destroying our health to more healthful choices.

For those who continue to suffer, especially after you have eaten or drank a highly sugared drink (alcohol) or after a meal or acidic ash causing food, taking a simple remedy like bicarbonate of soda (baking soda) in a small glass of water will relieve the burning almost immediately. Also using a couple teaspoons of apple cider vinegar in water is helpful for some people. But hopefully you will not need this after you have finished reading my book and put into practice my guidelines.

The Mystery Behind Alkaline/Acid Balance. The pH in your blood is tightly regulated by a complex system of buffers that are continuously at work to maintain your body to be more alkaline than acid. Actually the food that you eat does not directly affect the pH of your body as the body was designed to maintain its' balance.

So this is not a "simple" process of your diet affecting the alkaline/acid balance in your body.

To put it simply, pH is a measure of how acidic or alkaline a liquid is in your body. The liquids we areconcerned with, are of course, our body fluids. There are two main groups:

1. <u>Intracellular fluid</u> – is the fluid in all of your cells.

2. <u>Extracellular fluid</u> – is the fluid found outside of your cells. There are two types of these fluids: Plasma, your blood, and Interstitial fluid, which are the spaces that surround your tissue, i.e., fluids around your eyes, lymphatic system, joints, nervous system and that surrounding your cardiovascular, respiratory and abdominal cavities.

Additional Concerns. Acid reflux is not the only health problem as a result of the liquid in our body being too acid. Cancer is a major result of an acid environment. Experiments have shown that cancer cells cannot live in an alkaline environment. The more acidic we are, the more likely cancer cells will grow. One of the main causes of the cancer cells to grow is sugar. Yes, those candy bars you have to have every day, or that highly sugared Starbucks coffee you are addicted to contribute majorly to the growth of cancer cells. Does this sound too simple? It may, but our bodies were designed to work in a particular way and it is up to us to find out what it is that encourages good health, as simple as it may seem. So you see why I call acid reflux a symptom?

This is probably more information than you wanted to know, but bear with me as I am trying to make a very complex subject as simple as I know how, without over simplifying it.

Fluids In Our Bodies. Now how does the food we eat affect the fluids in our body? There are certain minerals in foods that, after they are metabolized, throw off alkaline or acid residues. When you ingest foods and liquids, the end products of digestion and assimilation of nutrients often results in an acid or alkaline-forming effect – the end products are referred to acid ash or alkaline ash. These residues are what determine our sickness or health.

There are other ways our bodies produce alkaline or acid waste. This is through our everyday metabolic activities.

According to Dr. Ben Kim, there are two main forces at work on a daily basis that can distrupt the pH of your body fluids (1) the acid forming effects of foods and liquids that you ingest, and (2) the acids that you generate through regular metabolic activities, but fortunately your body has mechanisms at work at all times to prevent these forces from shifting the pH of your blood.

These mechanisms are our buffering systems that are in place to prevent dietary, metabolic and other factors from pushing the pH of your blood outside of the healthy range of 7.35 to 7.45.

So why do we encourage you to "alkalize your blood," meaning you should eat plenty of foods that have an alkaline-forming effect on your system? The reason for making this suggestion is that the vast majority of highly processed foods - like white flour products and white sugar - have an acid-forming effect on your system, and if you spend years eating a poor diet that is mainly acid-forming, you will overwork some of the buffering systems mentioned above to a point where you create undesirable changes in your health. Dr. Ted Morter calls this "keeping your backup systems on red alert". When you keep your body on "red alert" because of an unhealthy acid diet for months or years, your system and organs become exhausted. An exhausted body cannot compete with disease. Eventually disease wins the game.

Other Concerns of an Acidic Environment. Another reason for being concerned with an over acidic body is we are over taxing of our bodies' buffering system, and interferes with the calcium in your bones and teeth. If your body system is regularly exposed to large quantities of acid-forming foods and liquids, such as animal products and canned drinks, your body will draw upon it's calcium phosphate reserves to supply your phosphate buffer system to neutralize the acid-forming effects of your diet. Over time, this may lead to structural weakness in your bones and teeth.

This is just one example of how your buffering systems can be over taxed to a point where you experience negative health consequences. Since your buffering systems have to work all the time anyway to neutralize the acids that are formed from everyday metabolic activities, it is your best interest to follow a diet that does not create unnecessary work for your buffering systems.

The Good & the Bad. Generally speaking most vegetables and fruits have an alkaline-forming effect on your body fluids.

Most grains, animal foods, and highly processed foods have an acid-forming effect on your body fluids.

Your health is best served by a good mix of nutrient-dense, alkaline and acid-forming foods; ideally, you want to eat more alkaline-forming foods than acid-forming foods to have the net acid and alkaline-forming effects of your diet match the slightly alkaline pH of your blood. If you have health issues related to an overabundance of acid residue from poor dietary practices over the years, you need to look at eating 90% alkaline, or even 100% alkaline, particularly if cancer is an issue. As I mentioned, cancer cells live and grow faster in an acid environment. And again, acid reflux is a result of eating too much acid forming foods. Also, keeping an alkaline balance helps your blood to be more oxygen rich.

Summary. So to sum this all up, the food we eat definitely has an effect on how alkaline/acid your body is because of the stress we put on our buffering system and yes, these foods do have an effect on how healthy we are and how well our bodies can fight disease. A recent study found that about 1 in 5 new cases of cancer in the US involves someone who has had the disease before. Does this tell you something? Unless we change what we eat and our lifestyle, our body will stay in an unhealthy state.

I have learned that using the pH strips to test your urine, can show the acid or alkaline residue in the body, but the test needs to be done several times a day. Your best test is how you feel and if disease is present in the body.

I will leave it up to you to check out the many sites where you can find detailed charts showing acid-forming and alkaline-forming foods. I only present this information for educating people about their own bodies and how to help maintain a healthy body. I do not claim that this information will prevent disease in any way. Do not stress out about this. Just be aware and try to eat as balanced a diet as you can.

Now on to the next chapter. Aren't you excited to find out what stronghold I am going to break you of? Let's venture on.

BALANCE 3

PART 1 – IMPORTANCE OF EATING CLEAN

"Today, more than 95% of all chronic disease is caused by food choices"

Mike Adams, Health Ranger

Clean Eating. You've probably heard of clean eating, but you may not know what it is exactly or how to go about cleaning up your diet! Eating clean is a good way to refresh your eating habits: it's about eating more of the best and healthiest options in each of the food groups-and eating less of the not-so-healthy ones. That means embracing foods like organic vegetables, fruits and healthy grains, plus healthy proteins and fats. It also means cutting back on refined grains, added sugars and unhealthy fats. It means eliminating processed foods, basically anything out of a can or box. Eating whole foods these days can be challenging, but once you read this book, you will have enough information to make the transition easier. But, since it does not entail counting calories or giving up whole food groups, it should be easy to follow. The health journey you are beginning should be considered a life-long change without an end date or return to previous unhealthy habits. It is simply changing the way you live and making choices today to maximize your health and effectively improve the quality of life.

The Basic Principles of Eating Clean

Eating clean involves not only choosing the right foods to eat but also avoiding all of the junk foods and processed foods that are so readily available. The keys to good health and proper nutrition are in the following principles.

- **Eat whole foods**: Whole foods are foods that haven't been tampered with, in the lab or the manufacturing plant. The foods you eat on this plan are straight from the farm: organic fruits and vegetables, certain whole grains, unsalted raw nuts, and seeds. This could also include following a raw food diet. On a raw food diet most of what you eat are plant based foods that are high in vitamins, minerals, fiber, phytochemicals and enzymes.

- **Avoid processed foods**: Processed foods are any food that has a label. A label means that more than one ingredient was used to make that food. It means changing the form of the natural food, for instance, removing the bran and germ from whole grains to create refined bread, removing the bran from rice and bleaching it to make it white, adding coloring to make it more appealing as in cheddar cheese. They actually add coloring to make yellow. Stick to the white cheeses. If you can't pronounce an ingredient on a label, don't put that food in your shopping basket.

- **Avoid GMOS**. A GMO (genetically modified organism) is the result of a laboratory process where genes from the DNA of one species are extracted and artificially forced into the genes of an unrelated plant or animal. The foreign genes may come from bacteria, viruses, insects, animals or even humans. Our food supply is over-processed, contaminated with multiple chemicals and compromised permanently by dangerous Genetically Modified Organisms (GMOs). At best, it lacks the nutritional potency necessary to support good health and sustain a species. See more on GMOs later.

- **Eliminate refined sugar**. Refined sugar provides nothing but calories. Other sweeteners can be used, but **do not make the mistake of substituting artificial sweeteners**. Good sugar substitutes are Xylitol and Stevia. With all the good foods you add to your diet, refined sugar really has very little place in the eating clean plan. See more later.

- **Eat five or six small meals a day**. By eating smaller meals throughout the day you can help rev up your metabolism and reduce the chance that you'll eat something not conducive to good health. When we are hungry this is when we stop for that McDonald's shake or fries. So always keep something healthy to snack on. Raw nuts, cut up raw veggies and fruit. Do not be taken by the trend to buy so called "healthy" snack bars that are loaded with sugar and other additives. There are many snack bars that are truly healthy, you just have to read labels. As you get used to eating healthy, your body will adjust and you will find your own personal way of spreading out your meals.

- **Prepare your own meals**. Instead of buying meals in a box, cook meals from scratch. That's not as hard as it sounds! Clean, whole foods need little preparation beyond chopping and sautéing to make satisfying, delicious meals your family will love. As a break from eating a heavy, cooked meal, I used to have a meal of fresh raw veggies. I would cut up green beans, carrots, celery, cucumbers, cherry tomatoes, and even raw potatoes. I would add a hard boiled egg for the protein. My children got used to eating raw vegetables. In fact, even when I was cooking vegetables for dinner, my children would ask for some of the raw veggies I was cooking.

- **Combine protein with carbs**. When you do snack or eat a meal, make sure that meal is balanced. For the most satisfaction from your diet, and so you'll be less tempted to eat junk food, combine protein with carbs or carbs and fat. This simple act will fuel your body and quash hunger pangs.

How Whole Foods and Eating Clean Help You Stay Healthy

What you eat really does have an effect on how you feel. Eating whole foods and avoiding junk food - a clean eating lifestyle can keep you healthy or help you regain your health if you haven't been well. Follow these precepts and you will have a better chance at living an active life:

- It's easier to maintain a healthy weight, which reduces the risk of several diseases.

- Eating a good variety of foods ensures you get adequate amounts of most essential nutrients.

- Relying on whole foods is the best way to get a good combination of micronutrients.

- Whole foods keep you satisfied longer so you're less tempted by junk foods.

- Foods high in micronutrients can help reduce cholesterol levels and regulate blood sugar.

- There are some nutrients we haven't yet identified that are present in whole foods but not in supplements.

- Whole foods help keep your digestive system regular.

- Eating a healthy diet makes you stronger so you can stay more active.

- Avoiding artificial ingredients keeps your cells strong so your body systems work efficiently.

- If you feel good, you're more likely to take care of yourself in other ways.

- Learn to read labels on everything. If you cannot pronounce an ingredient, do not buy it.

Spicing Up Your Meals When Eating Clean

Healthy food has an undeserved reputation for being boring or bland. Whole, fresh foods are actually delicious on their own, with no added seasoning. Unfortunately, many of us have been jaded by too much sodium, sugar, and additives in our food. But there are healthy ways to add flavor to clean foods Here are some herbs and spices you can use in your daily cooking:

- **Basil**: This bright-green delicate leaf contains flavonoids that act as powerful antioxidants. It's also high in vitamins A and K and has a good amount of potassium and manganese. You can grow basil plants on a sunny windowsill throughout the year or grow it in your garden and preserve it by freezing or drying it. Use peppery and minty basil in tomato sauces, salad dressings, pesto, sandwich spreads, soups, and chicken, beef, pork, and fish dishes.

- **Marjoram**: This fragrant herb contains many phytochemicals - including terpenes, which are anti-inflammatory - lutein, and beta carotene. Plus, it has lots of vitamin C and vitamin D. Marjoram is delicious in any dish made using beef and is perfect with vegetables like tomatoes, peas, carrots, and spinach. Together with bay leaf, parsley, thyme, and tarragon, it makes a bouquet garni to use in stews and soups.

- **Mint**: Mothers used to offer mint to kids for upset stomachs because it soothes an irritated GI tract. But did you know it may be a weapon against cancer, too? It contains a phytochemical called perillyl alcohol, which can stop the formation of some cancer cells. Mint is a good source of beta carotene, folate, and riboflavin. Use it in teas, in desserts, as part of a fruit salad or lettuce salad, or as a garnish for puddings.

- **Oregano**: Used in Italian dishes, this strong herb is a potent antioxidant with the phytochemicals lutein and beta carotene. It's a good source of iron, fiber, calcium, vitamin C, vitamin A, and omega-3 fatty acids. Who knew that spaghetti sauce could be so good for you? Add spicy and pepper oregano to salad dressings, soups, sauces, gravies, meat dishes, and pork recipes.

- **Parsley**: Do you ever wonder what's happened to the entire parsley garnish that has been left on plates in restaurants over the years? If only people knew then how healthy it really is! This mild and leafy herb is an excellent source of vitamin C, iron, calcium, and potassium. Plus, it's packed with flavonoids, which are strong antioxidants, and folate, which can help reduce the risk of heart disease. Use it in everything from salads as a leafy green to rice pilafs, grilled fish, and sauces and gravies.

- **Rosemary**: Rosemary contains terpenes, which slow down free radical development and stop inflammation. Terpenes may also block some estrogens, which cause breast cancer. Use this pungent and piney herb in soups, stews, meat, and chicken dishes. Chop some fresh rosemary to roast a chicken, cook with lamb or beef, or mix with olive oil for a dip for warm whole-wheat bread.

- **Sage**: Sage contains the flavonoid phytochemicals apigenin and luteolin and some phenolic acids that act as anti-inflammatory agents and antioxidants. Perhaps sage's most impressive effect may be against Alzheimer's disease by inhibiting the increase in AChE inhibitors. Its dusky, earthy aroma and flavor are delicious in classic turkey stuffing (as well as the turkey itself), spaghetti sauces, soups and stews, and frittatas and omelets.

- **Tarragon**: This herb tastes like licorice with a slightly sweet flavor and is delicious with chicken or fish. It's a great source of phytosterols and can reduce the stickiness of platelets in your blood. Tarragon is rich in beta carotene and potassium, too. Use it as a salad green or as part of a salad dressing or mix it with Greek yogurt to use as all appetizer dip.

- **Thyme**: This herb is a good source of vitamin K, manganese, and the monoterpene thymol, which has antibacterial properties and may help protect against tumor development. It's fresh, slightly minty, and lemony tasting, making it a great addition to everything from egg dishes to pear desserts to recipes featuring chicken and fish.

- **Cinnamon**: The aroma of cinnamon is one of the most enticing in cooking; just the smell can help improve brain function! It can also reduce blood sugar levels, LDL cholesterol, triglycerides, and overall cholesterol levels. Cinnamaldehyde, an organic compound in cinnamon (go figure!), prevents clumping of blood platelets, and other compounds in this spice are anti-inflammatory. Add cinnamon to coffee and tea, use it in desserts and curries, and sprinkle some on oatmeal for a great breakfast.

- **Cloves**: These flower buds are a great source of manganese and omega-3 fatty acids. They contain eugenol, which helps reduce toxicity from pollutants and prevent joint inflammation, and the flavonoids kaempferol and rhamnetin, which act as antioxidants. Cloves are a great addition to hot tea and coffee as well as many dessert recipes, including fruit compote and apple desserts.

- **Cumin**: This spice is rich in antioxidants, which may help reduce the risk of cancer. It also has iron and manganese, which help keep your immune system strong and healthy. Add cumin to Middle Eastern recipes, rice pilafs, stir-fried vegetables, and Tex-Mex dishes.

- **Nutmeg**: Nutmeg is rich in calcium, potassium, magnesium, phosphorus, and vitamins A and C. It can help reduce blood pressure, acts as an antioxidant, and has antifungal properties. The lacy covering on nutmeg is used to make mace. Keep a whole nutmeg in a tiny jar along with a mini rasp to grate it fresh into dishes with spinach, add it to hot tea, use it in curry powder, and add it to rice pudding and other desserts.

- **Turmeric**: This spice is one of the healthiest foods on the planet. Curcumin, a phytochemical in turmeric, can stop cancer cells from reproducing and spreading, slow Alzheimer's disease progression, and help control weight. In fact, researchers are currently studying curcumin as a cancer fighter, painkiller, and antiseptic. Turmeric gives foods a pretty yellow color and is an inexpensive substitute for saffron. Use it in Indian foods, egg salads, sauces, tea, and fish and chicken recipes.

- **Salt**: As far a health goes, salt has a bad reputation. According to a clinical research study reported in The Journal of Medicine, Vol.119, 3/2006, the authors of this study did not find any direct association of sodium with cardiovascular disease (CVD). In addition, this study noted that a reduced sodium diet leads to negative health issues. Sodium deficiency can occur when the body perspires heavily and a pattern of dehydration sets in This could lead to a rapid decrease in blood pressure. It could also lead to an alkaline/acid imbalance in your body.

- Some of the benefits of salt are: salt is needed for good digestion; improves metabolism; supports thyroid function; reduces stress hormones and is actually a natural antihistamine. The bad rap from salt comes from the overuse of salt in processed foods, not from the use at the dinner table or in cooking.

- The question is, what kind of salt should I be using? Should I buy these expensive natural salts? I would definitely eliminate boxed salt. It has been processed and bleached with even the smallest minerals destroyed. Sea salts, such as Himalayan, Celtic, Icelandic salts all still have their natural minerals intact. So my preference is to go the extra and buy one of the organic sea salts.

- **Pepper**: Incredibly popular black pepper, often referred to as "king of spice", is a well known spice since ancient times. The peppercorn pod is actually a berry from the pepper plant. Pepper stimulates the taste buds in such a way that an alert is sent to the stomach to increase hydrochloric acid secretion, thereby improving digestion. It is also noted to have antioxidant and antibacterial effects.

- There are many other spices you might like to try. Stretch your horizons and try something different the next time you prepare a meal.

Clean eating is not a new concept. In fact, chances are your grandparents never talked about "eating clean." Instead that is the way they ate because clean food, food that is simple, natural, unprocessed, and whole was what was available. In recent years those involved with health, fitness or nutrition from competitors to personal trainers and health conscious individuals have taken up the banner of practicing clean eating.

If you have never eaten this way before it may take some practice and some time to get 100% clean. Unprocessed, natural state foods have a different taste than frozen and processed foods. Your taste buds will go through an adjustment period. Give yourself time to adjust. Most recipes can be adapted to a clean eating lifestyle. Although it is less expensive to eat clean and nutritious foods, it does require more time in the kitchen planning and cooking meals. Once you get used to planning, it actually becomes natural and routine to shop and cook this way.

Some tips to help you on your way:

Clean out your pantry. We need not look any further than our pantries and refrigerators for the answer to today's obesity and health crises. The vast majority of pantries and refrigerators are overflowing with foods that promote disease and lack living foods that not only prevent disease, but also can reverse many of today's most dangerous degenerate diseases. Processed food in bags and boxes filled with white flour, white sugar, high-fructose corn syrup line the pantry shelves, while bottled high sugar juices, jams, meats, cheese, dairy and desserts fill our refrigerators. The first step in making a life-long dietary change is to purge your putty and refrigerator of unhealthy foods if you do not get rid of the package and canned food in your pantry, you will wind up using them. Start clean.

When you shop, shop with a list. Now that you have purged your kitchen, you are ready to purchase food that will strengthen, heal and regenerate your body. When you shop, shop with a list. This keeps you from buying things that do not belong with your new way of eating for your health. So many of us will go to the grocery store for a quick trip, without a list, and wind up buying a dozen items you had no intention of buying. I know, I am guilty of this.

<u>Nothing white</u>. No sugar, no white flour (bread, pasta, etc.), no white rice. If it is white, and it is not a vegetable, do not eat it. As far as sugar goes, do not get into the trap of using artificial sweeteners! See my thoughts on artificial sweeteners. There are good sweeteners that can substitute for sugar such as xylitol and stevia. Some people recommend honey or agave. Stay away from agave, raw honey is ok occasionally or dark maple sugar.

<u>Healthy sources of Fats</u>. Be sure all fats you are consuming are from a healthy source. Fats such as olive oil, coconut oil (research the many health benefits of coconut oil) and nut oils are healthy fats. Organic, of course Avocados are an excellent source of healthy fats.

No Alcohol. This is a personal choice. If a glass of wine occasionally or a beer does not lead to more, this may fit for you. Even here you have a choice of buying organic.

Lots of Fruits & Vegetables. If you are serious about eating clean, buy only organic fruits & vegetables. See Part 3 on Organic.

Assortment of raw nuts and seeds-raw unsalted almonds are great, so are walnuts, pecans and chia seeds.

Clean Meats. Your source of animal protein is very important in eating clean. Grass feed, grass finished meats are more nutrient dense. Their flesh is less acid, which means they are more easily digested. Also free range chickens grown organically and eggs from free range chickens have much more flavor and contain no growth hormones.

Clean Fish. Fish is among the healthiest foods that we can eat. Fish contain good fats and protein. They supply us with heart and brain healthy omega 3 fats. But again, buyer beware. There are bad fish and good fish. Bad fish are most those fish that contain high amounts of mercury and anti-biotics. The larger fish like sword, mackerel, grouper eat smaller fish and which increases the amount of mercury in their flesh. Also you want to eat wild caught fish, and stay away from farmed fish. For example, farmed salmon is feed grain and fish parts. Salmon eat krill, which is what gives them their notable red color. Farmed salmon are given dye to give them their color.

Check the internet for the best fish to eat. But I will only buy wild caught fish.

Grains. Wheat is something I have eliminated. A lot of nutritionists recommend eating whole grains. I myself believe even whole grains are not healthy.

The wheat grain that is grown today is not the same as the grain of our grandparents. It has been so genetically modified our bodies do not even recognize it as food. You probably have heard of "wheat belly." Study this and you will see why whole grains that most bread products are baked from today are not a good choice. If you do want to eat wheat, just make sure it is organic whole wheat.

There's a whole world of grains that many people don't even realize are out there - each has a unique nutritive benefit, some are even gluten-free! Super grains pack fiber, protein, vitamins and minerals along with carbohydrates. And, of course, you do not need to have Celiac disease or be gluten sensitive to want to broaden your grain intake and diversify from wheat and corn. The US Dietary Guidelines recommend eating at least 6 servings a day of grains- so why not eat better grains that will do more for you? Some suggestions would be quinoa, millet and kamut, spelt and amaranth. Experiment, step out of the box, there is a lot to explore. Of course there is also brown rice, which is one of my favorite.

Most of all, give yourself time to adjust. As the old saying goes, Rome wasn't built in a day. This is not an overnight happening, this is a lifestyle change. It is tough to change, so be kind to yourself, and give it time. God created your body with the amazing ability to adapt when it is presented with new circumstances or environments. You can learn to not only tolerate, but actually enjoy foods that you may not like today.

So hopefully these tips will help you get started on your way for you and your family to eat clean. Onward to new horizons.

BALANCE 3

PART 2 – GREEN IS CLEAN

"It is bizarre that the produce manager is more important to my children's health than the pediatrician"

Meryl Streep

"**Eat your Vegetables**" - we have all heard this statement many times from our mothers as well as our doctors and health professionals. That quote has never been more true than today. With the amount of free radicals that enter our bodies daily and the stress levels put on us, diet is more important today than ever before.

Advantage of Green Food. The phyto-nutrients found in green foods are full of vital anti-oxidants and plant-based vitamins and minerals. Green foods is a general term introduced decades ago that is now becoming a household term. It can refer to products that are made from fruit and vegetable extracts, often sold as capsules, tablets, wafers or powders. Taking these supplements can be the nutritional equivalent of eating the nine fresh servings of fruits and vegetables that we should consume daily, but often do not.

Common ingredients in green foods include blue-green algae, chlorella, wheat grass, activated barley grass, kelp, kamut, and spirulina.

Green foods supplements can support most bodily functions, boost energy levels, and eliminate toxins such as heavy metals, which can weaken our tissues and lead to disease over time.

Studies have also shown the antioxidant-rich chlorella to help reduce high blood pressure, lower LDL or "bad" cholesterol, accelerate wound healing, improve general immune functions, and help with colitis and fibromyalgia.

There are other nutritional benefits of green foods, as well. They have been shown to support cellular metabolism, and because they are naturally alkaline, they help to neutralize excess acidity which is a common problem with the standard American diet.

Aesthetically, green foods provide benefits such as better looking skin, hair and nails. Some research suggests that green foods can even delay the natural effects of aging.

Although the last decade has seen a lot of green foods supplements enter into the market, we have found certain criteria that we feel are very important in making an educated decision when choosing a greens product.

Organic and Non-GMO. First and foremost, the product should be organic and non-GMO. Also, excessive heat can degrade a product, so it is important to get your greens in a raw or un-processed state. Lastly, watch out for products made with fillers and binders. These things have nothing to do with greens and are often used because they are less expensive.

Digestion. Another notable benefit of green foods has to do with digestion. When taken, as we said before, green superfood powder also works as an effective alkalizer, helping to reduce the acidity in your body. All disease thrives in an acidic environment, so easy ways to support alkalinity are valuable as a preventative measure to help you avoid developing disease in the first place. I go into more depth on this in **Balance 2**. As they say, prevention is the best cure so by increasing regularity and keeping our digestive tract operating efficiently, we can dramatically increase our chances of being a healthy you.

Optimum health involves providing our bodies with the best possible nutrients for maintaining cellular wellness and function. Greens products should be part of everyone's foundation for good health, and come in a variety of sources for multiple use. One of the easiest ways to integrate green superfood powders into your routine, is in the form of a green smoothie. They can be mixed with juices, water, or blended into a smoothie with apples, bananas, berries, and/or protein powders for a complete meal replacement.

Price could be a deterrent. If the price seems steep when purchasing your green super powder, consider that one tablespoon of this powder can give you your greens for the day. Also, consider the alternative, the cost involved with getting sick. this would be a lot more costly. Of course fresh is best, but for people on the move, sometimes a powder is a fast, convenient way to get some dense nutrition and vitamins. Supplementing an already healthy diet with a daily scoop of green powder is a recipe for vibrant health.

I like using my super greens in this way to supplement eating my green leafy vegetables. I use my green drink on the go, it is convenient and gives me energy. Also for someone like my husband who avoids eating vegetables at all costs, he will drink his green drink when I mix it for him. Also it is great for children. It is much easier to mix up a super green drink and have them drink it, it tastes so good, then arguing with them to "eat your vegetables." But they do need to learn to love vegetables. My son Donny said he learned to love vegetables because he said I always made them sound so good and because of the variety of vegetables I encouraged them to eat.

When you try your supper greens, as I stated before, just make sure the super greens you are drinking are organic and non-GMO. If you want more info on super green powder check out this website www.mypurium.com

So by now you have been successful in "eating clean", going "green", now it is time to move on to the next step in enhancing your life style to a healthy you. There is more!

BALANCE 3

PART 3 – EATING ORGANIC

"You (God) satisfy me more than the richest of foods"

Psalm 63:5

Chemicals in Our Food. Eating organically grown foods is the only way to avoid the cocktail of chemical poisons present in commercially grown food. More than 600 active chemicals are registered for agricultural use in America, to the tune of billions of pounds annually. The average application equates to about 16 pounds of chemical pesticides per person every year. Many of these chemicals were approved by the Environmental Protection Agency (EPA) before extensive diet testing.

The National Academy of Sciences reports that 90% of the chemicals applied to foods have not been tested for long-term health effects before being deemed "safe." Further, the FDA tests only 1% of foods for pesticide residue. The most dangerous and toxic pesticides require special testing methods, which are rarely if ever employed by the FDA.

Regardless of diet, organic foods are a smart priority. Opting for organic foods is an effectual choice for personal and planetary health. Buying organically grown food-free of harmful chemicals, bursting with more nutrition, taste, and sustainable sustenance-is a direct vote for immediate health and the hopeful future of generations to come.

Benefit from more nutrients. Organically grown foods have more nutrients-vitamins, minerals, enzymes, and micronutrients-than commercially grown foods because the soil is managed and nourished with sustainable practices by responsible standards. The Journal of Alternative and Complementary Medicine conducted a review of 41 published studies comparing the nutritional value of organically grown and conventionally grown fruits, vegetables, and grains and concluded that there are significantly more of several nutrients in organic foods crops.

Further, the study verifies that five servings of organically grown vegetables (such as lettuce, spinach, carrots, potatoes, and cabbage) provide an adequate allowance of vitamin C, whereas the same number of servings of conventionally grown vegetables do not. On average, organically grown foods provide 21.1% more iron (than their conventional counterparts); 27% more vitamin C; 29.3% more magnesium; 13.6% more phosphorus.

Enjoy better taste. Try it! Organically grown foods generally taste better because nourished, well balanced soil produces healthy, strong plants. This is especially true with heirloom varieties, which are cultivated for taste over appearance.

Avoid GMO. Genetically engineered (GE) food and genetically modified organisms (GMO) are contaminating our food supply at an alarming rate, with repercussions beyond understanding. GMO foods do not have to be labeled in America. Because organically grown food cannot be genetically modified in any way, choosing organic is the only way to be sure that foods that have been genetically engineered stay out of your diet.

What is GMO? Genetic engineering is different from traditional crossbreeding. GMO stands for "genetically modified organism". In engineering six major GMO crops, soy, corn, cotton, canola, sugar beets and alfalfa, a gene from a virus or bacteria was forced into the DNA of the plants. Derivatives such as soy lecithin, soy protein, high-fructose corn syrup and sugar (unless labeled as cane sugar) are in the vast majority of processed foods. The pesticide giant, Monsanto and other pesticide producing companies, are now injecting pesticides into the seeds of these plants and others. The food companies are under siege from consumers' growing demand for natural and less industrially produced food. We need to stand behind our beliefs and let our Congress men know we want GMO labeling on food that has been modified. This is the norm in Europe.

Many US consumers mistakenly believe that the US Food & Drug Administration (FDA) approves GMO crops only after careful study. Instead, the agency claimed it was not aware of any significant difference from other food crops and declared safety testing unnecessary. In reality, according to FDA documents later made public in a lawsuit, the consensus among FDA scientists was the GMOs were different and dangerous and needed rigorous, long-term testing to prevent allergies, toxins, new diseases and nutritional problems.

Why is Roundup, Monsanto's weed killer for GMO crops so toxic.

Monsanto portrays Roundup as a benevolent herbicide. This is a lie. Glyphosate, its active patented ingredient, alters biochemical pathways in the body. Scientists such as Anthony Samsel and Stephanie Seneff have linked glyphosate to numerous diseases and disorders, including cancer, heart disease. diabetes, gluten sensitivity,

Alzheimer's, Parkinson's, depression, autism and reproductive disorders. In March, the World Health Organization (WHO) declared it a probable carcinogen.

The problem with this practice, is the label on these foods containing these altered ingredients, do not have to be listed on the labels. So the consumer is unaware that the can of corn, or the crackers with high fructose corn syrup in them, contain these dangerous ingredients. There are currently nine GMO food crops, which now include zucchini, yellow squash and papaya grown in Hawaii or China. Any packaged grocery product not labeled "Non-GMO" or "Organic" is likely to contain at least one GMO; this includes meat and dairy products from animals that have eaten GM feed.

Moms Across America is a national coalition of unstoppable Moms committed to empowering millions to educate themselves about GMOs and relative pesticides and to get GMOs labeled. Consumers have a right to know and sixty-four other countries do label GMO products. Why not US? Monsanto a billion dollar giant corporation has deep pockets and stands to lose lots of money if, indeed, products were to be labeled. They were able, just recently, to get a bill defeated in California by pouring millions of dollars into this campaign. Monsanto is also injecting seeds with pesticides and they have convinced the FDA to make it illegal for farmers to use heritage seeds in their plantings. Farmers are being arrested because they insist on using seeds from crops not injected with these dangerous pesticides. This is a good reason to support your small local organic farmers, as so far, they are being left alone.

The solution. Buy Organic and food labeled "Non-GMO." By buying organic, non-GMO foods, food companies will feel the loss of profits and remove the GMOs. This is already happening. You can read daily of companies eliminating the GMOs from their products (even McDonald's) NonGMOShoppingGuide. com is a reliable source that lists about 30,000 non-GMO products. Supporting and shopping at your local health food stores will ensure that you are getting organic, non-GMO foods. I supported our local health food store forty years ago when the first co-op health food store opened in Cocoa Beach. None of my friends understood why I would pay a little extra for food when it was cheaper to shop in the big box stores.

Conventional meat and dairy are the highest risk foods for contamination by harmful substances. More than 90% of the pesticides Americans consume are found in the fat and tissue of meat and dairy products. The EPA reports that a majority of pesticide intake comes from meat, poultry, fish, eggs, and dairy products because these foods are all high on the food chain. For instance, a large fish that eats a smaller fish that eats even smaller fish accumulates all of the toxins of the chain, especially in fatty tissue. Cows, chickens, and pigs are fed animal parts, by-products, fish meal, and grains that are heavily and collectively laden with toxins and chemicals. Lower-fat animal products are less dangerous, as toxins and chemicals are accumulated and concentrated in fatty tissue.

Antibiotics, drugs, and growth hormones are also directly passed into fish, meat and dairy products. Tens of millions of pounds of antibiotics are used in animal feed every year. The union of concerned scientists estimates that roughly 70% of antibiotics produced in the United States are fed to animals for nontherapeutic purposes. US farmers have been giving sex hormones and growth hormones to cattle to artificially increase the amount of meat and milk the cattle produce without requiring extra feed. The hormones fed to cows cannot be broken down, even at high temperatures. Therefore they remain in complete form and pass directly into the consumer's diet when meat is eaten.

Hormone supplementation is the biggest concern with beef, dairy products, and farmed fish. In the United States, the jury is still out. However, Europe's scientific community agrees that there is no acceptably safe level for daily intake of any of the hormones currently used in the United States and has subsequently banned all growth hormones.

Switching to Organic. Sales of organic food grew by 11% nationwide in 2014, according to the Organic Trade Association (OTA). The growth was seen in all regions, with the highest sales penetrations in New England and the Pacific Northwest. Other regions are not far behind.

The OTA said organic foods account for 4% of total US food sales, but acreage devoted to organic farming is less than 1% of the cropland. This is changing. This is part of the "revolution". Even big box stores like Publix and Walmart in our area are opting to have more selections of organic produce and meats.

Buy Organic! So doesn't it make sense to buy organic. What used to be on the fringe of society is now becoming more mainstream as more and more consumers are becoming aware of the benefits of buying organic. What about you. This is a choice you will need to make.

Make good choices. One way to navigate through all the conflicting health information is to make nutrition choices based on sound principles, which can act as solid guideline when you are confronted with all sorts of varying opinions. Here are three which work well.

The best and healthiest food comes from a farm or field, not a factory. Do you want to eat plastic food or plastic oils? Avoid any synthetic ingredients or additives. Period.

Eat food in its whole form as much as possible. So much of our food is overly processed and refined. Important nutrients have been stripped away, transforming food that was one healthy into junk food, or non-food.

Eat food in its raw form as much as possible.

What about you. These are choices you will need to make. The choices you make with your pocketbook will determine the outcome of the revolution towards a healthier you!

BALANCE 3

PART 4 – THE CASE AGAINST AFTIFICIAL SWEETENERS

"Research has shown that artificial sweeteners promote insulin resistance &related health problems, just like sugar does"

Dr. Mercola

Positive Instruction. In writing this book I did not plan on getting into controversial subjects. My objective was to walk someone through some positive steps in changing their outlook on getting to be that healthy you. But as you read in **Balance 1 - My Story**, artificial sweeteners have been a part of my "revolution" for a very long time.

If you can't convince them, confuse them - This is a quote attributed to President Harry Truman and I think this is so appropriate for today's deceptive advertising. Despite copious scientific evidence of harm, artificial sweeteners, for example, are promoted in advertising and by "experts" in general, as safe because they "pass through your body undigested." This is a not true. False advertising, promotion by big pharma and big corporations has convinced the pubic that what is known by scientific proof, indeed, artificial sweeteners are harmful, the general population turns their head and ignores what is an established truth.

Avoid artificial sweeteners! A long with the introduction of aspartame many other artificial sweeteners have come about, mainly because the uninformed public has bought into the falsehood that using these sweeteners are "healthier" than using sugar! So as long as the public buys into this untruth, manufactures will continue to use it and call it "healthy." The following is a small list of what you should avoid.

- Aspartame (NutraSweet)

- Sucralose (Splenda)

- Saccharin (SweetN' Low)

- Acesulfame Potassium

- Noeotame

Aspartame is perhaps the most dangerous of the lot. At least it is the most widely used and has the most reports of adverse effects. There are hundreds of scientific studies demonstrating its harmful effects. Do a study for yourself.

This fanatical mother strikes again! When my children were in middle school, I was able to convince the principal to shut down the drink machines in the school cafeteria. I asked them to quit supplying the machines with soda and diet sodas. And by providing scientific research which showed the negative effects of aspartame on young children's brain and showing the effect of sugar on children's behavior, the school did quit supplying the drink machines with soda and diet sodas. My daughter today still remembers the empty soda machines. She thinks they had some kind of tape around them so the kids could not buy the sodas. That lasted only about one semester. Other mothers were outraged that their children were denied the opportunity to buy soda from the drink machines. I not only stand by my beliefs, but I act on them too. I have also tried to educate my friends on the negative consequences of drinking diet drinks. When it is my time to host my card game group (Bridge) I will not serve diet drinks. Some of my friends asked why I did not serve them, I just said that I had no desire to poison my friends in my home!

Public Beware! What is so sad about all this, is the fact that artificial sweeteners also appear to cause many of the same health effects associated with high sugar consumption. Most recently, a report published in the journal *Trends In Endocrinology & Metabolism* highlighted the fact that diet soda drinkers suffer the same exact health problems as those who opt for regular soda, including excessive weight gain, type 2 diabetes, cardiovascular disease and stroke. So the very reason anyone would consider using diet instead of sugar sweeteners has no basis in fact. Anyone using them would get the same problems as using regular sugar and expose themselves to the well documented risks of artificial sweeteners!

Just recently our local Florida Today Newspaper published an article on "How Safe Are Artificial Sweeteners?" It touted the so called benefits of these sweeteners concluding there was no harm and that they "weren't even absorbed by the body." I had to respond and did write a letter to the editor showing research to the contrary. Here is some of the research I quoted.

- *Preventative Medicine 1986* -- "...users were significantly more likely to gain weight."

- *Purdue University* ... found saccharin consumption can lead to weight gain.

- *Journal of the American Dietetic Assoc.* "...there is no evidence that artificial sweeteners use was associated with a decrease in their overall sugar intake" They also found in subsequent research that their use contributed to an increase in type 2 diabetes.

- *Duke University...* "a link between the consumption of artificial sweeteners, gut bacteria and obesity has been charted."

- *Journal of Biology & Medicine 2010...* "increasing evidence suggests that artificial sweeteners do not activate the food reward pathways in the same fashion as natural sugars...thereby increasing the craving for sugar and sugar dependence.

There are many more studies. I was very pleased when the Florida Today did publish my rebuttal.

Natural Sweeteners. I am also going to burst your bubble of what you have been told about some "all natural" sweeteners. Natural sweeteners such as honey and agave may seem like a healthier choice, but not only are they loaded with fructose, many are also highly processed. In that regard, you are not gaining a thing. The health effects will be the same, since it is the fructose that causes the harm.

- **Agave Syrup** - Agave syrup can be considered as harmful as high fructose corn syrup because it is a higher fructose than any commercial sweetener. What is worse, most agave "nectar" or agave "syrup" is nothing more than a laboratory-generated super condensed fructose syrup, devoid of virtually all nutrient values. So be very careful when you buy agave syrup.

- **Honey** - Honey is also high in fructose, but contrary to agave, it is completely natural in its raw form and has many health benefits when used in moderation. But again beware of much of the honey sold in your grocery stores. Grade A honey is highly processed and of poor quality. Buy from your local health food store and you should buy local harvested honey from local bee keepers.

- **High Fructose Corn Syrup** - I was a little confused as to whether to place this under the "natural sweeteners" or "artificial sweeteners." The goal of the corn industry is to confuse the public by calling their product natural "corn sugar." Quoting Dr. Mark Hyman, "This is like calling tobacco in cigarettes natural herbal medicine." The makers of high fructose corn syrup (HFCS) are telling you there is no difference between natural cane sugar and HFCS. It is true that over consumption of sugar in any form is harmful, but with the increase of HFCS in our food we are consuming enormous amounts of fructose. When you start reading labels, you will be shocked at the number of processed foods that contain the HFCS. HFCS and sugar are not biochemically the same and are not processed by the body the same way. It is an industrial food. So buyer beware, check labels, better yet, do not buy anything in a box or can.

- **Cane Sugar**. Of course, I need to mention just regular old sugar. Life was much easier when our only choice was just plain old table sugar. But now, the choices vary so much it is hard to know which way to turn. Cane sugar comes from the natural sugar cane plant. My husband grew up in Florida where sugar cane was grown. As kids they used to chew on the sugar cane stalks.

You see a lot of "health products" sweetened with organic cane sugar. Do not be deceived, this is just sugar whether organically grown or whether it is "raw." The way the sugar is processed may be different, but the composition is the same. The difference is that when sugar is refined they strip the sugar cane plant of all its' natural components and is processed into what we know as table sugar. This means they take the sucrose out of its natural balance and consequently our body does process it differently. When sucrose, sugar, is part of the whole food it acts like a food in our body, entering our system calmly, breaking down slowly and providing a range of nutrients in addition to energy.

Conclusion - Raw sugar is probably the lesser of these evils but be mindful of your sugar consumption and as with all things, everything in moderation. After all, sugar does provide the body with energy.

- **Black Strap Molasses**. This is basically what has been stripped from the sugar cane plant. A lot of people classify this as a super food. Black strap molasses encompasses most of the nutritious parts of the sugar cane plant. It contains Vitamin B6, manganese, magnesium, potassium, iron and selenium. The vitamins and minerals occur in natural proportions since it comes directly from the sugar cane plant. But again, it is high on the glucose chart.

Effects of fructose on your system. What does fructose do to your body?

- It tricks your body into gaining weight! Does this surprise you? It does this by fooling your metabolism, as it turns off your body's appetite-control system.

- It activates a key enzyme that causes cells to store fat.

- It rapidly leads to weight gain and abdominal obesity, decreased HDL, increased LDL, elevated triglycerides, elevated blood sugar, and high blood pressure.

- Sugar is broken down in your liver just like alcohol, and produces many of the side effects of chronic alcohol use, including non-alcoholic fatty liver disease.

- And over time, leads to insulin resistance, which is not only an underlying factor of type 2 diabetes and heart disease, but also many cancers. Remember cancer cells feed on sugar.

What is a safe alternative? The safest alternative, as I said before, is to cut down on your sugar consumption. Eating lots of sugar is an addiction, just like any other addiction. You consume high amounts of sugar, i.e., craving those donuts in the morning along with your highly sweetened coffee, having that candy bar in the afternoon to give you "energy", needing to have dessert after a good meal. These are behaviors that lead to your sugar "addiction." This may be the hardest accomplishment in all that I have suggested in eating healthy. I know that, but taking baby steps will lead you to manage these addictions.

Three of the best sugar substitutes, and yes there are some alternatives, Stevia, Lo Han Guo and Xylitol.

- Stevia - is a highly sweet herb derived from the leaf of the South American plant. When we, in the "crazy health nut" community, first became aware of stevia, it could not be sold in the US as a food. I remember having to buy it as a cosmetic and mix it myself. Imagine trying to tell someone to mix this cosmetic into your tea or coffee and sav it is a sweetener? I guess that is why we were called "nuts!" But it is completelysafe in its natural form. But again, "buyer beware" one of the big corporations have found a way to screw this up too. Truvia is not the natural stevia plant, it has some added ingredients. So the best place to buy your stevia is at a health food store. The drawback with stevia is that is does have an objectionable after taste for some people.

- Lo Han Guo - is another natural sweetener similar to stevia, but is a bit more expensive and not as easy to find. In China, the Lo Han fruit has been used as a sweetener for centuries, and it is about 200 times sweeter than sugar.

- Xylitol - this is a sugar alcohol and the reason it is recommended is the fact that it does not get completely absorbed into your body and does not have an effect on your blood sugar. There are other sugar alcohol products on the market, but the Xylitol is rated as the best. This is my choice. But even xylitol can have its side effects, too much can cause diarrhea. Also Xylitol does combat bacteria, so it is my choice in the toothpaste I use (of course, no fluorides).

So what next, take this as one of your "revolutions" and see if we can't get the trend of putting aspartame and artificial sweeteners in everything out there reversed. One of biggest shocks pertaining to as partame, was when they started putting it in gum, along with the sugar! How crazy is that. The only way we can get changes made is if we stop buying these offending products. When they can feel it in their pockets, than maybe change will come about.

So continue to forge forward, there is more!

BALANCE 4

IMPORTANCE OF DETOXIFYING YOUR ENVIRONMENT

"By cleaning your body on a regular basis and eliminating as many toxins as possible from your environment, your body can begin to heal itself, prevent disease, and become stronger and more resilient than you ever dreamed possible"

Dr. Edward, Global Healing Center

Let's face it - we live in a toxic world! Recent years have brought reports of heavy metals such as lead in products, and the subsequent ongoing avalanche of product recalls, this is just the tip of the iceberg. For example, municipal tap water in most cases is contaminated with heavy metals. Automobile exhaust fumes spew them out constantly into the air that we breathe. Produce that is not organic contains heavy metals. The truth is, it is impossible to completely avoid exposure to heavy metals.

But the news is not all bad. As a result of these developments, we are becoming more aware of our toxic environment and are taking steps to change that and lessen the toxins on the planet and on our bodies. We are recycling more and making wiser choices in our daily lives - hopefully you have already made the switch to organic grown produce, or started using household products that contain minimal amounts of toxic chemicals and heavy metals.

Dangers of toxins in our environment. Toxins can wreak havoc on your body, your biochemistry, your cellular health, and the environment. These endocrine disruptors can mess with the hormones that keep your metabolism running smoothly. But ditching the processed, chemical laden foods in your diet (which is a good start) is not enough, you have to remove toxins from your HOME, too. From household cleaning products to cosmetics and cooking tools, limiting your exposure to household toxins will help reduce hormonal threats, reboot your metabolism, and make you feel like your best.

I realize this is no easy task - and may take time and effort, especially if you are the homemaker. Children are especially sensitive to the chemicals that surround us. Even when you are pregnant these chemicals can cross the placenta to the fetus and accumulate, it can cause mental retardation, brain damage, cerebral palsy, blindness, seizures and inability to speak in young children who have been exposed to these chemicals in the uterus.

According to some research being exposed to these toxins may cause criminal behavior as an adult.

As a start on your journey, I am listing eight areas to consider as you give your living space an eco-makeover.

1. **Eliminate cans**. Many food and beverages are lined with Bisphenol-A (BPA), a chemical linked to breast cancer and other health concerns. I hope by now you are not using canned processed food, so that this has already been eliminated from your pantry.

2. **Plastics can be our enemy**. Many chemicals of concern are found in plastic. There are many unsuspecting items in your home you have not even thought about, starting in your kids toy bin, aka plastic toys. Also PVC, for example, plastic shower curtains. Also by now, I hope you have eliminated your plastic storage containers and substituted glass. Especially how you carry your water with you. If you have to buy a bottle of water to take with you, NEVER drink out of it if it has been left in your car overnight.

   Another reason to avoid plastics is the fact that they are suspected to be the cause of male infertility and erectile dysfunction, ED.

   A study from the University of Mexico conducted in 2023 found microscopic particles in male testicles. The study found that microscopic plastic particles can penetrate blood testicles barrier.

   Plastics are xenoestrogens. Xenoestrogen is an estrogen hormone. Men are ingesting and being exposed to high level of estrogen, a mostly female hormone in large amounts, leading to male impotence, reduced sperm production and erectile dysfunction. ED is becoming an epidemic in the 40 to 80 male population.

It is actually very easy to eliminate or reduce this problem i.e., eliminate the use of plastics in storing our food; avoid using any plastics, such as cups, utensils and other plastic materials. Drinking hot coffee from a Styrofoam cups is a major way of ingesting plastic.

3. **Beware of what is under your kitchen sink** - more on this later in the article. Choose green cleaning products to drastically reduce indoor air pollution. Because cleaning product formulas are currently government protected trade secrets, consumers cannot get the full list of chemicals by reading ingredient lists in an effort to avoid harmful chemicals. We can look out for danger labels and warnings.

4. **No matter what you read, cleaning is not disinfecting.** The dirtiest thing in any home is your own two hands. Still, many cleaning products, personal care products, and even socks, now contain antibacterial agents, added to make consumers feel safe. It is a false safety as these antibacterials can lead to antibiotic resistance. Even the American Medical Association says it is prudent to avoid anything that says it is antibacterial. Soap and water gets the job done without harming you, your kids, or the environment - or creating super bugs. It pains me when I see mothers using these antibacterial products on their children. It also lowers their immune systems by lowering their natural resistance to bacteria in their natural environment. We are trying to all live like the "boy in the bubble" (you have to be a certain age to know about this) and keep all the germs away from ourselves and our kids. It cannot be done.

5. **Now for the big ones that you may not be aware of.** If your house was built before 1978, check it for lead paint. Also it is advised not to use anything in your home that

was painted prior to the advent of removing lead from paint in the late 1970s.

6. **Personal Care products**. This is a tough one for most women. We have our favorite products and we hate to give them up, but do this one product at a time. Personal care products like makeup, lotions, and even shampoo do contain chemicals that have been linked to everything from reproductive complications to cancer. Choose natural, clean versions from companies that do not use things like parabens, and a whole host of petroleum-derived ingredients.

7. **Pesticides are very dangerous**. If you eat organic to minimize ingesting pesticide residue, why spray poison in your kitchen or garden? Products like boric acid is great for eliminating roaches, ants and silverfish. Say goodbye to your exterminator and rely on natural pest solutions combined with preventative measures instead. Pesticides have been linked to a range of health problems, including asthma, hyperactivity and behavior problems, cancer, learning disabilities, reproductive disorders, and compromised brain development. Removing your shoes at the door is a good habit to get into and will decrease the amount of pesticides your track into your home.

8. **More is Not Better**. Buying less stuff you bring into your home, the fewer chances you have for bringing in potentially harmful substances.

Choosing safe products is so important but the waters can be hard to navigate at first. Here are some tips to choosing safe products.

Ingredients Matter. I know I mentioned that cleaning products do not have to list everything in them, but there are ingredients that you must avoid.

- Ammonia. Toxic when inhaled, swallowed or touched.

- Antibacterial's & Disinfectants. I went into detail about these in paragraphs above.

- Chlorine Bleach. It is a very strong, corrosive & irritating to both lungs & eyes.

- Petroleum Solvents. Many ingredients are derived from petroleum by products.

- Phosphates. These are harmful to aquatic life & mostly found in laundry detergents.

- Phthalates. These can come in the form of fragrances. Avoid scents altogether.

- Butyl Glycol, Ethylene Glycol, Monobutyl. Very dangerous to our nervous system, liver & kidneys.

Also, do not be fooled if the label says "Natural;" "Non-Toxic" or even "Eco-Friendly." This is a marketing tool that is being used on everything. The "Natural" label is at present, one of the biggest hoaxes being perpetrated on the American public. Read the ingredients!

Now that I have gotten you all upset about your cleaning products. There are several alternatives that you can make yourself. The following is a list of easy to find items that will be great substitutes for all your household chores. Know them, use them, save money and you will be thankful for the decrease in toxic matter in your home.

- **Baking soda** is great for cleaning so many things. From hard water to pet messes and smells, baking soda is a hero. Combine it with a little water to scrub up just about anything to a nice shine. Add to vinegar or dish soap for super strength to clean tile, pots and pans, carpet, tubs, toilets and even stains on clothing. Also, baking soda and coconut oil make a great toothpaste.

- **Vinegar** is good for just about anything. I have used both white vinegar and apple cider vinegar in cleaning. I like white vinegar for general cleaning. I will take the peelings off of a grapefruit or orange, let them soak in about a 1/2 cup of white vinegar for a couple of days, add about a cup of water to that mixture and you will have a wonderful smelling and general cleaning agent for very little cost. You can add an essential oil to the vinegar and water mixture instead of the peelings.

Apple cider vinegar is great for cleaning toilets (plus a little baking soda to foam up), showers, sinks and other tough water/ mildew spots (and oh, it is a fabulous hair conditioner, something I used when I was growing up). Mix up your own all purpose and glass cleaners. Add it to your laundry in the rinse cycle for a great fabric softener. It will also take the odor from your clothes. Even put it in your dishwasher's rinse aid compartment. Vinegar is amazing.

- **Castile Soap** is a gentile soap made from vegetable oil (often olive oil) as opposed to animal fat or synthetics. This stuff is great for use in general cleaning, laundry, body wash, and even shampoo.

- **Air fresheners** and candles are not part of the cleaning process, but we often use them to cover unpleasant odors or just as a soothing, calming atmosphere. The fragrances used in these products are not what you think. The gingerbread holiday candle, the cinnamon candle, the vanilla scent air fresheners are not what we think they are and usually do not contain these wonderful herbs, but actually contain dangerous benzene chemicals that have serious side effects. I for one, get a terrible headache if I am someplace where they are burning a vanilla scented candle. Many people have more serious respiratory side effects. As an alternative look for soy-based candles, and essential oils for these uses.

Now I know there are those of you out there that would maybe start to use these home-made items, but many out there would rather buy ready made safe, toxic free cleaners. There is an organization that tests and recommends safe, toxic free products. It is The Environmental Working Group, a non-profit organization focused on environment and public health. Their website is www.ewg.org. You can find the products they have tested and rated.

I for one like the products that Evolv Health provides (www. evolvhealth.com). They take the guess work out of buying cleaning products and are committed to making the home a healthier and safer place by supplying products that do not contain toxic chemicals.

Also you can buy safe cleaning products at your local health food stores. Some of your big box stores are carrying safer products, but again, "buyer beware." Just because the word "natural" is on the label, does not mean there are no harmful chemicals in the product.

Happy, healthy cleaning!

BALANCE 5

FILTERED WATER – OUR MOST IMPORTANT NUTRIENT

"Water Sustains all"

Thales of Miletus 600BC

Water Our Most Important Nutrient. The human body requires more water than any other nutrient. Virtually everything that happens in our bodies requires the assistance of H2O to take place. That means without sufficient amounts of water, life processes suffer.

Unfortunately, many of us do not hydrate adequately. That causes us to experience lack of energy, inability to focus and concentrate, memory problems, sluggish fat metabolism, an impaired immune system, abnormal bowel function, and lack of ability to efficiently eliminate toxins.

Water retention in the body is often the result of dehydration. That may seem counter-intuitive, but when the body does not have the water it needs, it perceives that as a threat to survival and holds onto as much as it can. Water is stored in the spaces outside the cells, and shows up as swollen hands, feet, ankles, legs, etc. The following are health issues caused by lack of good hydration.

- Constipation is often caused by inadequate water intake. When the body does not get the water it needs, it siphons from the colon. When adequate water is consumed, normal bowel function normally resumes.

- Lack of water is the No. 1 cause of fatigue. Simply drinking enough water throughout the day will significantly increase your energy level if you are dehydrated.

- Headaches and minor joint and muscle discomfort are often caused by dehydration. Proper hydration keeps your muscles and joints lubricated so that you are less likely to get cramps and sprains.

- Fat metabolism depends upon water. If you are trying to lose weight, be sure to drink plenty of water to maximize your fat burning capacity. I have often found that many of my overweight friends do not drink nearly enough water. After they become fully hydrated, they often comment about how much easier it is to lose weight.

When we are dehydrated, our natural thirst and hunger sensing mechanisms become distorted. When your body becomes well hydrated, your natural thirst returns and hunger begins to diminish.

Athletes know very well how dehydration can affect performance. As little as a 2 percent water loss (through sweat or dehydration) result in a noticeable decline in strength and power, precision, speed and endurance.

How Much Is Enough. So, with all that being said, how much is enough? You may have heard that eight cups a day is the recommended amount. That is a good ballpark figure. It is true that our bodies extract water from the foods and other liquids we consume, but that was accounted for when the guidelines were established. Most of us require an average of eight cups per day in addition to that contained in our food.

If you want to be more specific for your own individual water requirement use this formula: consume 1/2 ounce of water for every pound of body weight. As you gain or lose weight, your water requirement changes accordingly. It may seem like a lot of water at first, but will quickly adjust and will soon begin to experience the benefits.

To reiterate some of the points I have made, and also add some pointers, I have compiled the following list:

- 75% of Americans are chronically dehydrated.

- In 37% of Americans, the thirst mechanism is so weak that it is mistaken for hunger.

- Even mild dehydration will slow down one's metabolism.

- One glass of water will shut down midnight hunger pangs for 100% of the dieter's studies in a University of Washington study.

- Lack of Water, the #1 trigger of daytime fatigue.

- Preliminary research indicates that 8-10 glasses of water a day could significantly ease back and joint pain for up to 80% of suffers.

- A mere 2% drop in body water can trigger fuzzy short-term memory, trouble with basic math, and difficulty focusing on the computer screen or on a printed page.

- Drinking just 5 glasses of water daily decreases the risk of colon cancer by 45%, plus it can slash the risk of breast cancer by 79%, and one is 50% less likely to develop bladder cancer.

What Kind of Water Should I Drink. It is common knowledge that most water sources are now polluted, but there is tremendous confusion about what kind of drinking water is the most health promoting, and what kind of home water treatment produces the best drinking water.

Pure, Living Water. Of course, what you ideally want is pure water - water that is clean, balanced, and healthful. Some of the most healthful waters in the world are that which emerge from mountain springs. This mountain spring water is "structured" in a way that is not really understood. I know when I was growing up no one walked around with a bottle of water. I believe that our water then was "structured" to give us what we needed to hydrate our bodies. With all the efforts to give us "clean" water we have gone so far from what is natural, to water that is devoid of all the minerals that our body needs to hydrate. This was "living water". This is living in the same way that fresh, raw, organic food feeds our bodies to be strong and healthy.

How do we get that "living" water? Spring water coming out of a mountain spring is at this time the only source of this "living" water. I remember when I was in Brazil, the family that I was staying with would go a few miles to a place where there was a natural little water fall, take their bottles and fill them to bring home to use for drinking and cooking. Of course, spring water needs to come from deep aquifers that have not been contaminated. But where in this country could we actually find such a source? There is a website, www.findaspring.com where they have identified the locations of these natural springs. Check this website, it has some very interesting information. Even living in Florida there are natural springs where you can obtain spring water.

Here is a list of the types of water available to you.

- Purified Water. Water that is physically processed to remove impurities (i.e., distillation, deionization, reverse osmosis, carbon filtration, etc.).

- Distilled Water. Water that is boiled and evaporated away from its dissolved minerals, and then the vapor is condensed.

- Bottled Water. This water is typically from a spring or has gone through reverse osmosis before it is bottled. However, 40% of bottled water is regular tape water that may or may not have gone through any additional filtering. This industry is very loosely regulated. Plus, the chemicals that leach out of the water's plastic packages are also highly toxic.

- Alkaline Water. Water that has been separated into alkaline and acid fractions using electrolysis, which takes advantage of the naturally occurring electric charges found in the magnesium and calcium ions; in the drinking water industry.

- Deionized or demineralized water. Water in which the mineral ions (salts, such as sodium, calcium, iron, copper, chloride and bromide) have been removed by exposing it to electrically charged resins that attract and bind to the salts.

- Hard and soft water. Hard water containing an appreciable quantity of dissolved mineral; soft water is treated water in which the only ion is sodium.

- Well Water. There are many areas in this country that well water is the best water to drink. Well water can contain all the natural minerals found in the earth. My experience with well water is drinking the water that my daughter and her family drink from a well in South Georgia. It is always cool and tastes like real water. My other experience is from growing up in Florida where salt intrusion into our well was causing the water to not be consumable.

What Should I Drink. I am not here to tell what type of water filtration you should buy. You need to do your own research and decide what you are willing to spend and how much filtration you want. Just be sure if you are going to use a filtration system, that it has a multi-layer filter, not just a simple carbon filter. Do not be fooled by some of the cheap pitcher filtering systems, they really do not accomplish what needs to be done to make your water pure. There are some pitchers that have multi layered filters that do an excellent job. But, I do know, you need to do something about your drinking water. Municipal drinking water is highly contaminated with dangerous chemicals. These chemicals have been added to make you think you are drinking "safe" water. To name a couple, chlorine and fluoride. These two chemicals alone, should never be consumed. Not only dangerous to consume, but they are polluting our soil.

Fluoridation. Fluoride has been banned in 97% of Western Europe. Research from the UK's University of Kent has concluded that fluoridation of municipal water supplies may be more harmful than helpful, because the reduction in dental cavities from fluoride is due primarily from its topical application instead of ingestion. It was never meant to be consumed. Published in the Scientific World Journal the review which covered 92 studies and scientific papers, concludes that early research showing a reduction of children's tooth decay from municipal water fluoridation was flawed (are we surprised?) and did not adequately measure the potential harm from higher fluoride consumption and that overconsumption is associated with cognitive impairment, thyroid issues, higher fracture risk, dental fluorosis (mottling of enamel) and enzyme disruption.

Negative Effect of Fluoride.

In the last two decades, studies have suggested a different problem: a link between fluoride and brain development. Researchers are finding a negative effect on developing fetuses and very young children who ingest water with baby formula. Studies showed fluoride could impact neurochemistry cell function in brain regions responsible for learning, memory, executive function and behavior. (See my book "Brain Power" where I examine in length the effects on children's brains and fluoride.")

The researchers also found clear evidence for increased risk of uterine and bladder cancers in areas where municipal water was fluoridated. It is highly toxic to us and much more to our children. Because it has a negative impact on neurochemistry cell function, it could effect neurodevelopment disorders such as Alzheimer disease.

Bottom line, Fluoride is an unwanted byproduct of aluminum, fertilizer, and iron ore manufacturing. Fluoride is an industrial waste and extremely toxic.

Chlorine. According to the US Council of Environmental Quality, the cancer risk to people who drink chlorinated water is 93% higher than among those whose water does not contain chlorine. Drinking chlorinated water on a daily basis may cause some of these effects.

- Heat Attacks
- Tiredness, Dizziness or headaches
- Eye, Sinus, Throat Irritation
- Low Sperm Count in Men
- Miscarriages in Women
- Skin Rashes
- Liver Problems
- Kidney Problems
- A Weakened Immune System

The truth is, the water we use in and around our homes is far from the fresh, pure resource you might assume.

If Fluoride and Chlorine are so toxic, why haven't the government authorities done anything about it. Over the last 30 years a growing body of research has shown that these chemicals are very harmful to your health, however organizations like the Chemical Manufacturers Association have a serious well-funded interest in maintaining status quo. Even the EPA (Environmental Protection Agency) has been influenced to down grade the contamination level for chlorine. They used to have a maximum contaminant level goal of zero for chloroform in drinking water. They listed it as a probable human carcinogen. That was changed.

These are just some of the harmful chemicals found in our drinking water. As I stated above, many countertop and faucet water filters that are so widely available in the market place are totally inadequate. These are basically carbon water filters and the majority of them are ineffective in removing dangerous contaminates such as arsenic, bacteria, chromium, fluoride, microbes, nitrates, perchlorate, uranium and human viruses that can cause illness and even death. Our bodies cannot process these foreign substances.

This is as far as my recommendation for water filtration will go. It is up to you to research and decide which is best for you and your family.

Is all this information overload? I hope not, as I stated before, moderation is the key. You don't have to eat the whole enchilada at one time, change takes time.

BALANCE 6

FOOD AS OUR MEDICINE – THE COLOR PALATE

"Health is a relationship between you and your body"

Terri Guillemets

Simple Solution. This may seem to be too simple, but by making it simple it is easier to incorporate healthy eating into your everyday lives. I did not write this booklet to complicate people lives, but to make it easy to follow a few steps that could change your life and those of your family. I have known about the color palette of eating for years, but just recently it has become more predominate in the "healthy" gurus mantras. Do not discount it as too simple, but embrace it and you will find that as you get used to paying attention to the color palette of food, you will be more attuned to eating more of a variety of food.

"Eat a rainbow of colors often," Core Performance founder Mark Verstegen is fond of saying-and with good reason - "Eating a variety of colorful food provides vitamins, minerals, and antioxidants to nourish your body that cannot be replicated in a supplement."

Different colored foods play different roles in the body. Aim for at least three colors at every meal and two servings of fruit and three servings of vegetables over the course of the day.

Every meal should include colorful fruits and vegetables because of their fiber and nutrient densities. Proteins and carbs will most likely be brown, beige, or white. Add veggies like red peppers, carrots, and green beans to get your color quotient up.

Colorful Foods by the Numbers - 500 Eating three colors each night at dinner will add up to over 500 servings of vegetables over 6 months.

Red Foods - Packed with phytochemicals like lycopene and anthocyanins, red foods help increase heart and circulatory health, improve memory, support urinary tract health, and decrease the risk of certain types of cancers. Try these red foods:

- Cherries - This delicious fruit is high in antioxidants that have been shown to protect against heart disease, diabetes, and arthritis. A rich source of antioxidants, tart cherries also help reduce inflammation in the body and relieve pain from gout and arthritis.

- Cranberries - High in antioxidants and proanthocyanidins, cranberries have been shown to prevent bacteria from adhering to the urinary tract wall and reduce inflammation in the body.

- Red bell peppers - Bell peppers are low in calories and fat and high in vitamin C and fiber. Eating bell peppers (do not eat green bell peppers, as these are not ripe and could cause some digestive disturbances in some people) has been linked to increased immunity, improved digestion, lower cholesterol, and a decreased risk of colon cancer.

- Tomatoes - High in the antioxidant lycopene, tomatoes have been shown to help reduce damage to our cells and decrease the risk of cardiovascular disease and diabetes.

- Beets - This low calorie veggie is high in fiber, folate, and vitamins A, C, and K. Beets have been shown to optimize digestive health, decrease inflammation, and help fight heart disease.

Other Red Foods - Other delicious red foods include strawberries, raspberries, watermelon, pink grapefruit, pomegranate, red kidney beans, red apples, red grapes, red pears, radishes, radicchio, red onions, red potatoes, and rhubarb.

Orange Foods - Orange foods are high in antioxidants such as vitamin C, carotenoids, and bioflavonoids. Eating orange foods has been linked to skin and eye health, increased immunity, decreased risk of cancer, and a healthy heart. A few of our favorite orange foods include:

- **Carrots** - Carrots are high in vitamin A, which helps maintain the integrity of the skin, and beta carotene, which has been associated with boosting the immune system and potentially reducing the chances of skin cancer.

- **Oranges** - This fruit is high in vitamin A and C, which has been linked to increased immunity, heart health, and healthier skin. Also high in magnesium and fiber, oranges can help strengthen bones and improve digestion. Do not be mistaken that by drinking commercial orange juice in a carton or bottle you are getting the same nutrition as eating a whole orange, you are not! Once the orange juice is extracted the juice starts losing its vitamin A and C, especially when exposed to light. What you are drinking when you buy commercial orange juice is sugar water!

- **Sweet potatoes** - Often touted as one of the healthiest veggies we can eat, sweet potatoes are high in fiber, vitamins A and C, iron, and antioxidants. Eating sweet potatoes has been shown to promote healthy skin, increased immunity, and a decreased risk of cancer.

- **Peaches** - High in vitamin A, C, E, K, and fiber, peaches have been shown to help prevent cellular damage, promote healthier digestion, reduce inflammation in the body, and help reduce your risk of cancer.

Other Orange Foods - A few other orange foods to try include apricots, cantaloupe, Cape gooseberries, golden kiwifruit, mangoes, nectarines, papayas, persimmons, tangerines, butternut squash, and rutabagas.

Yellow Foods - Pineapple, yellow peppers, corn, star fruit, and other yellow foods contain nutrients that promote good digestion and optimal brain function. High in alpha- and beta-carotenes, yellow foods have also been linked to increased immunity, a decreased risk of some cancers, and healthy eyes and skin. Grab these yellow foods on your next shopping trip:

- **Pineapple** - Cholesterol and fat-free, pineapple is high in bromelain, an enzyme that helps regulate and neutralize body fluids and aids in digestion. Its high vitamin C content has also been linked to decrease in heart disease, cancer, cataracts, and stroke.

- **Yellow peppers** - High in vitamin C and A, yellow peppers have been linked to increased immune system and healthy skin. Yellow peppers are also high in carotenoids, which help protect from heart disease.

- **Star fruit** - Carambola, or more commonly known as start fruit, is high in high in vitamin C and calcium. This fruit has been linked to increased immunity, bone health, and muscle contractions.

Other Yellow Foods - Try some of the other delicious yellow foods like yellow apples, yellow figs, grapefruit, golden kiwifruit, lemon, yellow pears, yellow watermelon, yellow beets, yellow tomatoes, and yellow winter squash.

Green Foods - Green fruits and vegetables contain varying amounts of potent phytochemicals such as lutein and indoles. Benefits include a lower risk of some cancers, improved eye health, rejuvenated musculature and bone, and strong teeth. Stock up on these healthy green foods:

- **Broccoli** - High in calcium and iron, this veggie has been linked to stronger teeth, bones, and muscles, and a decreased risk of cancer.

- **Spinach** - This leafy green is high in antioxidants and vitamin K, which helps strength bones.

- **Kiwi** - Kiwi is high in folate, vitamin E, and glutathione, which all help decrease the risk of heart disease and promote optimal overall health.

- **Kale** - Probably the most important of the green vegetables, but most overlooked. Kale actually is high in calcium and other important nutrients.

Other Green Foods - Other healthy green foods include avocados, green apples, green grapes, honeydew, limes, pears, artichokes, arugula, asparagus, broccoli rabe, Brussels sprouts, Chinese cabbage, green beans, green cabbage, celery, chayote squash, cucumbers, endives, leafy greens, leeks, lettuce, green onions, peas, snow peas, sugar snap peas, watercress, and zucchini.

Blue/Purple Foods - These colorful foods get their bright hue from anthocyanins, which have been linked with antioxidants and anti-aging properties in the body. Blue and purple foods help promote bone health, and have been shown to lower the risk of some cancers, improve memory, and increase urinary-tract health. The main benefit of blue and purple foods is increased circulation and microcirculation. A few of our favorite blue/purple foods are:

- **Blueberries** - Blueberries are high in fiber (2.4 g per 2/3 cup), vitamin E and C, and antioxidants. Eating blueberries has been linked to improved cholesterol, increased urinary-tract health, and a boost in brain activity.

- **Blackberries** - These nutrient-packed berries are high in fiber, vitamin K (promotes calcium absorption and bone health), and high in antioxidants that improve overall health. Research has also linked blackberries to increased immunity, improved heart health, lower cholesterol, and decreased cancer risk.

- **Plums** - Plums are high in vitamin B, which helps metabolize carbohydrates, proteins, and fat. High in vitamin K, plums also help promote bone health.

- **Eggplant** - In addition to being high in fiber (8 percent of your daily needs), eggplant is also high in vitamin C, calcium, and phosphorus which promote strong bones and teeth.

Other Blue/Purple Foods - Other blue and purple foods to try are black currants, dried plums, elderberries, purple figs, purple grapes, raisins, purple asparagus, purple cabbage, purple carrots, black salsify, purple-fleshed potatoes, and purple Belgian endive.

White Foods - While many white foods are refined, like white bread and white rice, there are a lot of white foods that are packed with nutrients. White fruits and veggies have been linked to lower cholesterol, decreased blood pressure, and a lower risk of heart disease. The key benefit of white foods is increased immunity. Eating white foods helps enhance the immune system, the lymph systems, and aids in cellular recovery. Here are a few of our go-to white foods and their specific benefits:

- **Garlic** - In the same family as chives and onions, this powerful, potent food has been linked to heart health and decreased cancer risk. Garlic also has anti-microbial compounds.

- **Onions** - In addition to having powerful sulfur-bearing compounds that work as anti-microbial agents (similar to garlic), onions have also been shown to help lower blood sugar levels and improve heart health by lowering blood pressure and cholesterol. Onions are also high in the flavonoid quercetin, which has been linked to cell protection and slower tumor growth.

• **Cauliflower** - High in powerful antioxidants such as manganese and vitamin C. One cup of cauliflower has 52 mg of vitamin C, compared to 64 mg in a medium orange. This healthy food has also been linked to increased immunity.

Other White Foods - A few other healthy white foods include ginger, turnips, and jicama, white corn, turnips, shallots, white potatoes, parsnips, mushrooms, kohlrabi, Jerusalem artichoke, white peaches, and white nectarines.

And to make sure you are getting the most out of your fruits and vegetables, they need to be organic and non-GMO.

Getting Into A Rut. We get into ruts with our eating. It is time to step out and try some of the wonderful fruits and vegetables God has provided for us.

Eating what is in Season. Eat what is in season. Isn't this what our grandparents did on the farm? Avoid buying imported fruits and vegetables from other countries. You are best insured of getting organic non-GMO if you shop your local organic farmer. There are farms that offer memberships and they deliver to you fresh, in season fruits and vegetables.

7 Steps to A Healthy You. I hope you are now on the road to a healthy lifestyle. It will change your life. Now on to the core of it all.

BALANCE 7

TAKE ACTION!

PART 1 – CLEANSE YOUR BODY

"So whether you eat or drink or whatever you do, do it all for the glory of God"

1 Corinthians 10:31

A Personal Cleanse. Now that you have read through my book, and have taken the steps to change your lifestyle, I would suggest you start your lifestyle change with a personal cleanse. If you set the pace, your family will follow. But, of course before you start your cleanse, check with your doctor or health care professional. Doing a cleanse has been said to help unleash the natural healing power of your body by ridding it of built up toxins.

10 Day Cleanse. You can start with a 10 day cleanse. A cleanse is not a fast, so don't panic. By doing a 10 day cleanse it will be the beginning of a new, healthier you. After a cleanse you will be astounded at how your body feels. You will feel cleaner, your skin will look healthier, your taste buds will come alive and your metabolism will be heightened and many of your cravings will be gone. After a cleanse many of the harmful toxins that were stored in your fat layer will be gone (so will that belly fat). You will feel amazing.

In helping you along, the 10 day cleanse I recommend is found at www.puriumcorp.com. My family has used the super green shake, a whole raw, organic, nonGMO concentrated green food, and followed the cleanse with great success. Not only women like the cleanse, but men too, as you can eat some food with the cleanse. There are other concentrated green super foods on the market, but I have found this is the tastiest with superior quality control. You always have to be aware of any products that are not organic or nonGMO, and that contain fillers. Also for a great video on why we should be eating super green foods, watch on YouTube.com the video "Purium Farm to Family."

For an optimal super green cleanse experience, make sure you have the free time to reflect and able to rest. You can do this even if you are working. You just have to do more planning. Do not do a cleanse during an emotional intense time or during a major life transition. Do not start a cleanse if a birthday party is coming up or any event where food is the major part. Do not sabotage your cleanse even before you start. Set yourself up for success, ask you friends and family to support you or even do a cleanse with you. It is sometimes easier to do a cleanse with your husband to keep him on track. Also set yourself up for success for your cleanse by eating light 3 days before your cleanse. Get in the habit of eating only organic fresh fruits and vegetables and drink at least 8 glasses of water a day. But if you have been faithful and have read the other chapters in my book, all this should be old hat to you.

Set an intention for your super green cleanse. An intention is a commitment to changing a part of your life that no longer serves you. What is it you want to accomplish with your cleanse. Detoxing and losing some unwanted pounds is always a good intention and committing to a healthier life style for you and your family should be your ultimate goal. I wish you success on your road to a healthy you!

But there is more, be sure and read Balance 7 - Part 2, before you start your cleanse, it will help make it easier to move forward with your new healthy life style.

BALANCE 7

PART 2 – CLEANSE YOUR MIND

"Dear friend, I pray that you may enjoy good health and that all may go well with you…"

3 John 1:2

Thoughts Equal Actions. So now am I going to tell you to throw all I have said out the door? Heavens no! But this **Balance** is sometimes the most difficult to change. If you have spent a lifetime of thinking negative about your health, or seeing yourself as a fat little kid or living with a chronic disease, changing this one aspect of your personality is really going to be a challenge. The Bible teaches us that our thoughts are the determining factor which controls our actions. Proverbs 23:7 states, "For as he thinketh in his heart, so he is."

Our Thoughts Are Powerful. You do not have to think about everything that comes into your head. You can choose what to think about. Most people do not even think about what they are thinking about (Joyce Meyer). It is your own thoughts that make you feel the way you are feeling. You can have negative thoughts that will make you feel depressed. You can have uplifiting thoughts that will make you feel joyful. You can choose what you think about. This is pretty amazing. Have you ever thought about your thoughts this way?

What has this got to do with becoming a healthy you? No one can consistently perform differently than the way they think; therefore, we cannot change our actions without changing our thinking. It is not just what we think about that needs changing, but we must change our thought process. So many people have been conditioned into believing that the mind and body are separate things. There is never a time when the mind isn't influencing the body and vice versa.

Our Words. Words are not simply sounds caused by air pressing through larynx. Words have real power. God spoke the world into being by the power of His words. Words do more than convey information. The power of our words can actually destroy one's spirit. How do you respond to someone who asks you "how are you today?" Do you respond in the negative, "oh, I am feeling okay, but I have..." You are taking ownership of any malady if you continually complain about some minor or major health challenge you are facing. I am not making light of someone who is sick, I am just asking that you speak more encouraging words. The writer of Proverbs tells us, "the tongue has the power of life and death, and those who love it will eat of its' fruit." Are your words filled with hate or love, bitterness or blessing, complaining or compliments, or love and victory? Like any tool at our disposal, words can help us if we just are more careful what we speak.

Stress Affects Our Health. Stress can be positive, keeping us alert and ready to avoid danger. Stress becomes negative when a person continually focuses on the negative aspects of their life and continually worries about what might happen. Most of the time when we worry about negative results in a situation, it never comes about. Worrying about it does not change it, action does. We need to live with peace not stress. Our peace is linked directly with what we think. This generation, like no other before us, is plugged into the world. Reading, listening, and watching the negative news, movies and books has brought about a generation of fearful people. We need to find that peace, the "peace that passes all understanding."

Encourage. Be an encourager. Encourage others and encourage yourself. Apostle Paul states in Colossians 4:6, "let your conversation be always full of grace, seasoned with salt, so that you may know how to answer everyone." And Praise God, I want to be a part of encouraging you and helping you be strong and of good courage.

So with these encouraging words, I pray that you take what I have written and become a more healthy you in mind and body. And that you and your family have "peace that passes all understanding." If you want to have that kind of peace and would like to know more, email me at ahealthyyou15@gmail. com.

"But the fruit of the Spirit is love, joy, peace, longsuffering, kindness, goodness, faithfulness, gentleness, self control, against such as these there is no law."

Galatians 5:22-23

TAKE CHARGE OF YOUR HEALTH!

Author, Wife, Mother & Holistic Advocate, Lu shares her amazing story of how she navigated the maze of health from an early age. She has been on a quest for many years, educating herself, and all who will listen, helping people live an informed and healthy lifestyle.

7 Steps to Nutritional Balance gives the reader an easy to navigate guideline to the choices available in the market place. The book exposes many of the misinformation and the lies the media and big pharmaceutical companies are using to confuse the average family, confusing even people that are in the know, who are making an effort to eat a healthy diet and live a healthy lifestyle. I pray that these comprehensive guidelines will lead you and your family down a path of health and wellness. Join our revolution to help bring about a change in the marketplace by making informed choices. Create your own revolution by breaking through old eating patterns and taking responsibility for designing your own eating plan. It can be done!

ABOUT THE AUTHOR

Lu has been a pioneer in the health and nutrition field for well over 50 years. She is a strong advocate in taking control over one's own health and passing this knowledge on to their families. Lu have four children and 11 grandchildren and 5 great grand children. She could retire and enjoy her grandchildren, but feels the need to continue to encourage others in the wellness field.

www.ingramcontent.com/pod-product-compliance
Lightning Source LLC
Chambersburg PA
CBHW050010040726
47599CB00014B/1314